Revision Notes for MRCPsych Paper 1

Sarah Jawad
MB ChB
CT3 in Psychiatry

Foreword by

Wendy Burn
Dean
Royal College of Psychiatrists

Radcliffe Publishing
London • New York

Radcliffe Publishing Ltd
33–41 Dallington Street
London
EC1V 0BB
United Kingdom

www.radcliffehealth.com

British Library Cataloguing in Publication Data

A catalogue record for this book is available from the British Library.

ISBN-13: 978 184619 972 1

The paper used for the text pages of this book is FSC® certified. FSC (The Forest Stewardship Council®) is an international network to promote responsible management of the world's forests.

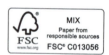

Typeset by Phoenix Photosetting, Chatham, Kent
Printed and bound by TJI Digital, Padstow, Cornwall

Contents

Foreword

It is my pleasure to provide a foreword to this book.

I have known Sarah since she was a first-year foundation trainee in psychiatry in Leeds and have always been very impressed by her enthusiasm, energy and commitment to psychiatry. It therefore does not surprise me that she has written a book so early in her career.

This book is designed as a revision aid for MRCPsych Paper 1 and is written in a concise, easy to read style. I am sure it will be helpful in supporting the learning needed to succeed in this examination.

Wendy Burn
Dean
Royal College of Psychiatrists
September 2012

About the author

Sarah Jawad graduated from Leeds University Medical School in 2008. Currently a Core Trainee 3 in Psychiatry in Leeds, she has a keen interest in liaison psychiatry and has already had experience of this subspecialty through her training rotations. She has also published several journal articles and presented these at regional, national and international levels. She is hoping to commence her Specialist Registrar Training in August 2013 with a view to progressing to a career in liaison psychiatry.

Acknowledgements

It would not have been possible to write this book without the continued support of my family Soheir, Sami, Ibrahim, Lena and Nadia. I am also extremely grateful to my partner Ravi whose love, encouragement, optimism and patience truly knows no bounds.

Chapter 1

History of psychiatry

Chapter 1
History of psychiatry

This part of the examination relies heavily on a good memory for names. There is no simple way to learn these, but dividing them into subsections with common themes can help make things more straightforward. These lists are by no means exhaustive, but provide a fairly extensive list of names that crop up regularly in membership exams and are worth your while trying to remember.

Early discredited theories

Hippocrates	Greek
	Father of medicine
	Coined the term 'hysteria'
	Notion of four humours
Galen	Roman
	Elaborated on Hippocrates' humoral theory

 A CLOSER look...

Hysteria

- Hippocratic view defined this as the 'movement of a women's uterus in her body'.

- Sydenham revised this definition and considered hysteria to harbour a psychological component.

Four humours

- Early theory proposing four main constituents of the human body: blood, yellow bile, black bile and phlegm.

- Imbalance of these 'humours' associated with disease or changes in temperament.

Anti-psychiatry

Cooper, David	Anti-psychiatry
Foucault	*Madness and Civilisation*
Laing	*The Divided Self*
Szasz	*The Myth of Mental Illness*

 A CLOSER look...

Anti-psychiatry movement

- Pivotal social movement.

- Proponents included David Cooper who coined the term 'anti-psychiatry' in the 1960s.

- Opposed traditional mental health practice from diagnostic labelling to subsequent treatment.

- Questioned increased medicalisation of psychiatry, considering mental illness a 'myth'.

- Criticised traditional psychiatric practice as too medicalised with lack of objective testing.

- Consensus that increasingly invasive procedures namely psychosurgery and seizure induction were harmful rather than useful.

- Criticism over what was perceived a violation of human rights to subject individuals to compulsory treatments.

Biological therapies

Bowden	Valproate
Cade	Lithium
Cerletti and Bini	Electroconvulsive treatment (ECT)
Charpentier	Chlorpromazine (synthesis)
Delay and Deniker	Chlorpromazine (treatment for psychosis)
Janssen	Haloperidol
Kane	Clozapine
Klaesi	Barbiturate coma therapy
Kline	Iproniazid, monoamine oxidase inhibitors (MAOIs)
Kline	Reserpine

 A CLOSER look...

Reserpine

- 1954

- Isolated from the *Rauwolfia Serpentina* plant.

- Its discovery shed light on the role of neurotransmitters dopamine, noradrenaline and serotonin in psychosis.

Kuhn	Imipramine
Meduna	Camphor-induced seizures
Moniz and Lima	Psychosurgery
Sakel	Insulin coma therapy
Sen and Bose	Reserpine
Sternbach	Chlordiazepoxide
Von Wagner Jauregg	Malarial treatment of general paralysis of insane

Psychological therapies

Adler	Individual psychology
Bannister	Repertory grid
Beck	Cognitive therapy
Berne	Transactional analysis
Ellis	Rational emotive therapy
Festinger	Cognitive dissonance
Freud	Psychoanalysis
Jacobson	Progressive muscular relaxation therapy
Janov	Primal therapy
Jung	Analytical psychology
Kelly	Personal construct theory
Klerman and Weissman	Interpersonal therapy
Linehan	Dialectical behaviour therapy
Mesmer	Hypnosis
Moreno	Psychodrama
Perls	Gestalt therapy
Rogers	Client-centred therapy
Wolpe	Systematic desensitisation

Group therapy

Bion	Group dynamics; basic assumptions (pairing, dependency, fight–flight)
Yalom	Group psychotherapy; curative factors (including cohesiveness, catharsis, instillation of hope, universality)
Foulkes	Group analysis (matrix)

Family therapy

Minuchin	Structural family therapy
Palazzoli	Systemic (Milan) family therapy
Haley	Strategic family therapy

Basic psychology and sociology

Ayllon and Azrin	Token economy
Bandura	Social learning theory
Bowlby	Attachment theory
Chomsky	Psycholinguistics
Durkheim	Sociological theory of suicide
Goffman	Total institutions
Jones, Maxwell	Therapeutic community
Klein, Melanie	Object relation theory
Maslow	Hierarchy of need
Mechanic	Ilness behaviour
Parsons	The sick role
Pavlov	Classical conditioning
Pilowsky	Abnormal illness behaviour
Seligman	Learned helplessness
Skinner	Operant conditioning
Watson, John	Behaviourism
Winnicott	Transitional object, good-enough mother

Psychosis

Bateson	Double-bind relationship
Bleuler	Schizophrenia
Crow	Type I and Type II syndromes of schizophrenia

Fromm Reichmann	Schizophrenogenic mother
Hecker	Hebephrenia
Kahlbaum	Catatonia
Kanner	Autism
Kasanin	Schizoaffective psychosis
Kraepelin	Dementia praecox
Langfeldt	Schizophreniform
Leonard	Cycloid psychoses
Liddle	Three-syndrome model of schizophrenia
Lidz	Marital schism/skew
Morel	Démence precoce
Schneider	First-rank symptoms
Wynne	Pseudohostility and pseudomutuality

Miscellaneous

Alexander, Franz	Psychosomatic medicine
Beard	Neurasthenia
Brown	Epidemiology
Cicero	Libido
Chomsky	Psycholinguistics
Cullen	Neuroses
Gockel	Psychology
Greisinger	Neuropsychiatry
Heinroth	Psychosomatic
Jaspers	General psychopathology
Meyer	Psychobiology
Pritchard	Moral insanity
Reil	Psychiatry

Rush	American psychiatry
Schneidman	Suicidology
Spitz	Anaclitic depression
Weyer	Modern psychiatry

Chapter 2

Aetiology and classification

Chapter 2
Aetiology and classification

Types of classification system

Familiarise yourself with the definitions below as they are commonly used to describe different approaches to classifying disease.

  A CLOSER look...

Descriptive. Does exactly what it says on the tin! Based on what observable factors make up the disease. Does not require the user to be aware of the aetiology of the disorder.

Operationalised. Includes specific criteria (exclusion and inclusion) that must be satisfied for a diagnosis to be made.

Atheoretical. As with descriptive, the atheoretical approach is based on observed factors (namely symptoms and signs exhibited by the patient) to make a diagnosis. It does not require a known cause to be identified.

Hierarchical. Based on the idea that one diagnosis can trump another. A good working example of this is the ICD-10. If an individual satisfies the criteria for an organic and a psychotic disorder, the organic diagnosis takes precedence over the psychotic disorder, particularly if the individual's psychotic symptoms are directly attributable to their physical health.

Categorical. The idea that a diagnosis is 'distinct'; either you have the disorder or you don't. Both ICD-10 and DSM-IV rely on a categorical approach.

> **Dimensional**. Opposite to categorical. Based on a continuum. Measurable on a scale. Examples of this are commonly numerical, such as weight or height measurements.

The 2 classification systems with which you should be familiar are ICD-10 (*International Classification of Diseases-10*) and DSM-IV (*Diagnostic and Statistical Manual of Mental Disorders*).

It is important to be aware of how these two systems compare. This has been highlighted 'A closer look...' below.

Differences between DSM-IV and ICD-10

The two main classification systems used to categorise mental and behavioural disorders are:

- *Diagnostic and Statistical Manual of Mental Disorders* (DSM-IV): An American classification

- *International Classification of Diseases* (ICD-10).

The box below highlights the key differences between these two systems, which are worthwhile remembering for membership exams.

 A CLOSER look...

Differences between ICD-10 and DSM-IV

ICD-10	DSM-IV
Produced in 1992	Produced in 1994
Psychiatric Classification dedicated to Chapter 5 of ICD-10. The remaining 20 chapters of ICD-10 allow for general medical classification.	Dedicated solely to psychiatric classification.
Four versions of ICD-10 exist: primary care version, clinical coding, research and diagnostic guidelines.	Single version for both clinical and research use.
Multi-axial. Three axes identified: mental disorder, disability and psychosocial functioning.	Multi-axial. Five axes identified: Axis 1 Major mental disorders Axis 2 Personality disorders Axis 3 Physical health conditions Axis 4 Psychosocial factors Axis 5 Global assessment of functioning

ICD-10 Classification of mental and behavioural disorders

A CLOSER look...

ICD-10 Chapter 5: Classification of mental and behavioural disorders

F00–F09	Organic syndromes
F10–F19	Mental and behavioural disorders due to substance misuse
F20–F29	Schizophrenia, schizotypal and delusional disorders
F30–F39	Affective (mood) disorders
F40–F49	Neurotic, stress-related and somatoform disorders
F50–F59	Behavioural disorders secondary to physiological disturbance
F60–69	Adult personality and behavioural disorders
F70–79	Mental retardation
F80–89	Disorders of psychological development
F90–99	Childhood and adolescence behavioural and emotional disorders

Classification and aetiology of specific disorders

This section does not cover all of the disorders outlined by ICD-10, but focuses purely on the disorders that commonly crop up in the MRCPsych Paper 1 and whose aetiological theories you are expected to be aware of.

Schizophrenia

Several subtypes of schizophrenia exist as demonstrated in the Closer look box.

A CLOSER look...

Subtypes of schizophrenia

- Simple schizophrenia. Largely negative symptoms with functional decline observed over a period of time. No positive symptoms evident.

- Catatonic schizophrenia. Psychomotor disturbances. Includes elective mutism and posturing.

- Hebephrenic schizophrenia. Largely changes in affect (mood) are observed. Disorganised thought and speech.

- Paranoid schizophrenia. Positive symptoms. Delusions and auditory hallucinations can dominate the picture.

- Undifferentiated. Does not appear to fall into a particular category.

ICD-10 and DSM-IV Subtypes

ICD-10 subtypes: Simple, catatonic, hebephrenic, paranoid, undifferentiated, post schizophrenic depression and residual.

DSM-IV subtypes: Catatonic, residual, undifferentiated, paranoid and disorganised.

NB Simple schizophrenia and post-schizophrenic depression are only recognised subtypes in ICD-10 and not DSM-IV.

Hebephrenia (defined in ICD-10) and disorganised (in DSM-IV) are different terms used to describe the same phenomenology.

Aetiology

Various theories of causality exist for schizophrenia.

(i) Genetic theory. Demonstrated by linkage/association studies. Family, twin and adoption studies also support a possible biological causation for schizophrenia.

A CLOSER look...

Genetic theories

- The following genes have been implicated (to name but two): *6p24-22* (dysbindin) and *8p* (neuregulin)

- Greater concordance in identical twins (monozygotic) than non-identical twins (dizygotic).

- Predisposition to schizophrenia in the proband (the individual of interest) is dependent on their relation to affected family members.

(ii) Biochemical theory

A CLOSER look...

Biochemical theories

- Role of the neurotransmitter dopamine has been postulated. Suggests that an excess of dopamine can result in positive symptoms of schizophrenia. Demonstrated by amphetamine use which releases stored dopamine and can subsequently mimic the positive symptoms of schizophrenia. Antipsychotic medication are also shown to act on dopamine receptors, which implicates the role of the neurotransmitter.

- Role of the neurotransmitter serotonin. Demonstrated by LSD which acts on serotonin receptors (5HT2A/5HT2C) and can induce psychotic symptoms. Second-generation antipsychotics are also known to have effect on these receptors.

- Role of the neurotransmitter glutamate. Demonstrated by phencyclidine (PCP) which binds to glutamate receptors via a non-competitive antagonism mechanism. This mechanism induces psychotic symptoms.

(iii) Obstetric factors

Winter–spring births have been associated with increased risk of schizophrenia.

Other obstetric factors that have been implicated include pregnancy complications and contracting maternal influenza, typically in the second trimester.

(iv) Psychosocial factors

The following factors have been associated with increased risk:

- Urban birth and living.

- Cannabis use. Increases risk by two- or threefold.

- Increased incidence of life events.

- High levels of expressed emotion are associated with increased risk of relapse. This relates to the individual's family and relatives.

Mood (affective) disorders

Aetiology

Various theories of causality exist.

(i) Genetic theory. Demonstrated by linkage/association studies. Family, twin and Adoption studies also support a possible biological causation for affective disorders.

A CLOSER look...

Genetic theories

- Polymorphisms at the serotonin 5HT2C receptor have been implicated.

- Concordance rates are higher in monozygotic twins than dizygotic twins.

(ii) Biochemical theory

A CLOSER look...

Biochemical theories

- Role of the neurotransmitter dopamine has been postulated. Suggested by low levels of homovanillic acid (dopamine metabolite) in the cerebrospinal fluid (CSF) of depressed patients.

- Role of the neurotransmitter serotonin. Tryptophan (the serotonin precursor) is found in low levels in the CSF of depressed patients. There are also low levels of 5HIAA (serotonin metabolite) in this cohort of patients. The action of antidepressants in increasing serotonin uptake highlights the role of this neurotransmitter in the causality of depression.

(iii) Neuroendocrine Theories

A CLOSER look...

Neuroendocrine theories

- Role of the hypo–pituitary–adrenal (HPA) axis. Increased cortisol secretion. Depressed patients typically exhibit non-suppression on dexamethasone suppression testing.

- Role of thyroid. Blunted Thyroid-stimulating hormone (TSH) response to Thyroid-releasing hormone (TRH).

- Blunted growth hormone (GH) response to clonidine.

(iv) Psychosocial factors

Brown and Harris Study identified vulnerability factors for developing depression, particularly in women:

- Loss of mother before age of 11

- Lack of confidante or support

- Unemployed

- Three children under the age of 14

Adult personality disorders

Personality disorders identified by ICD-10 include the following:

- Paranoid

- Schizoid

- Antisocial

- Emotionally unstable (impulsive, borderline subtypes)

- Anxious (avoidant)

- Dependent

- Anankastic

DSM-IV categorises personality disorder further and organises them into three clusters: A, B and C.

 A CLOSER look...

DSM-IV personality disorders

- Cluster A referred to as 'odd and eccentric':

  - Paranoid

  - Schizoid

  - Schizotypal

- Cluster B referred to as 'erratic and dramatic':

  - Borderline

  - Dissocial

  - Histrionic

  - Narcissistic

- Cluster C referred to as 'anxious':

  - Dependent

  - Avoidant

  - Obsessive–compulsive disorder

If we look at the subcategories in further detail and consider the key components:

Paranoid	Mistrust. Flat affect. Suspicious of others.
Schizoid	Socially withdrawn. Difficulty in forming relationships. Insensitive. Emotionless. Unresponsive to feedback from others.

Schizotypal	Magical thinking. Eccentric. Isolated psychotic symptoms. More common in the relatives of schizophrenic individuals.
Borderline	Unstable relationships. Impulsive. Self mutilation. 'Chronically empty'. Abandonment fears.
Dissocial	Oblivious to thoughts and feelings of others. No remorse for actions. Rule-breaker. Difficulty in maintaining relationships.
Histrionic	Dramatic. Self-centred. Attention-seeker.
Narcissistic	Sense of self-importance. Demands attention. Intolerance to others.
Dependent	Poor self-confidence. Dependent on others. Would much rather others assume responsibility for them.
Avoidant	Socially withdrawn. Poor self-esteem. Finds social gatherings difficult. Fear of rejection or criticism.
Obsessive–compulsive	Strives for perfection. Difficulty delegating. Limited emotion towards others.

Note the differences between ICD-10 and DSM-IV classification of personality disorders.

A CLOSER look...

ICD-10	DSM-IV
Schizotypal disorder is *Not* classified under personality disorder in ICD-10. Instead it is classified with F20–29, Schizophrenia	Schizotypal disorder
Antisocial personality disorder	Dissocial personality disorder
Emotionally unstable personality (impulsive and borderline subtypes)	Borderline personality disorder
Narcissistic personality disorder does not exist in ICD-10	Narcissistic personality disorder
Anankastic personality disorder	Obsessive–compulsive personality disorder

Chapter 3

Diagnostic tools and rating scales

Chapter 3
Diagnostic tools and rating scales

Rating scales: depression

There are various scales used by medical professionals in diagnosing and assessing the severity of common psychiatric conditions. Other scales are useful in determining clinical response to appropriate psychotropic medication once initiated. Such scales can be administered directly to the patient for self-rating or are objective tools used by the clinician themselves. For ease of revision, we have subdivided scales into self-rated and observer-rated. Further details about each individual test are given in the Closer look box.

Self-rated:	Beck's Depression Inventory (BDI)
	Hospital and Anxiety Depression Scale (HADS)
	Zung Self-rating Scale (ZSRS)
Clinician-rated:	Hamilton Depression Rating Scale (HAM-D)
	Montgomery Asberg Depression Rating Scale (MADRS)

A CLOSER look...

Depression

- Becks Depression Inventory (BDI). Self-rated, 21 items. Each answer is scored on a scale of 0–3 with a total score of 63 possible. A score of >28 is indicative of a severe depression. Can be used by individuals aged 13 or above. Considers how the individual has been feeling over the last two weeks.

- Hospital Anxiety Depression Scale (HADS). Self-rated, 14 items. Each answer is scored on a scale of 0–3 with a total score of 42 possible. Seven items pertain to symptoms of anxiety and seven to symptoms of depression. A total score of 21 is possible for both anxiety and depression. Allows clinicians to detect anxiety and depression experienced by the patient by focusing on psychological symptoms and less on biological symptoms (namely sleep and appetite) that can be accounted for by an organic cause.

- Zung Self-rating Scale (ZSRS). Used in individuals with a pre-existing diagnosis of a depressive disorder to assess the severity of their current symptoms. Self-rated, 20 items divided up into 10 positively worded and 10 negatively worded statements. Each item is scored on a scale of 1–4. Assesses both biological (somatic) and psychological symptoms. A score of >70 is consistent with a severe depression.

- Hamilton Depression Rating Scale (HAM-D). Clinician-rated. Used in patients with a pre-existing diagnosis of depression. Allows clinicians to rate the severity of the current episode. It considers the two-week period prior to assessment. Two versions exist, one of which consists of 17 items and the other of 21. The patient is scored based on interview with the patient and observation so it can be a fairly lengthy assessment taking approximately 30 minutes to complete. A score of >20 is indicative of a moderate depression.

- Montgomery Asberg Depression Rating Scale (MADRS). Clinician-rated. Used in patients with a pre-existing diagnosis of depression. Allows clinicians to rate the severity of the current episode. This scale is also commonly used to assess response to treatment. An improvement in score is often consistent with good effect of the antidepressant commenced. The total score ranges from 0 to a possible 60.

Rating scales: bipolar affective disorder

The Young Mania Rating Scale (YMRS) is the assessment tool most frequently referred to in MRCPsych Examinations.

An 11-item questionnaire administered by the clinician (i.e. observer-rated). It allows clinicians to assess the severity of manic symptoms.

Covers various items including mood, sleep and irritability.

Rating scales: anxiety

Commonly used anxiety scales are highlighted in the Closer look box.

A CLOSER look...

Anxiety

- Hospital Anxiety and Depression Scale. This has already been mentioned above, 14-item questionnaire, Self-rated. Each answer is scored on a scale of 0–3 with a total score of 42 possible. Seven items pertain to symptoms of anxiety and seven items to symptoms of depression. A total score of 21 is possible for both anxiety and depression. Allows clinicians to detect anxiety and depression experienced by the patient by focusing on psychological symptoms and less on biological symptoms (namely sleep and appetite) that can be accounted for by an organic cause.

- State–Trait Anxiety Inventory (STAI). Self-report, two scales, 'State' and 'Trait' each of which consists of 20 items. There are four possible responses to each statement. It enables clinicians to distinguish whether the anxiety experienced by the patient is a 'state', i.e temporary, or whether it is a long-standing (baseline) anxiety, namely a 'trait'. Straightforward to complete.

- Hamilton Anxiety Scale (HAS). Clinician-rated, 14 items. Used in patients with a pre-existing diagnosis of anxiety. Enables clinicians to rate the severity of anxiety. Each item is scored from 0–4. A score of 25–30 is indicative of a moderate–severe anxiety. Used widely in clinical and research trials.

Rating scales: schizophrenia

 ## A CLOSER look...

Schizophrenia

- Positive and Negative Syndrome Scale (PANSS). Clinician-rated. Time-consuming: can take up to 45 minutes to complete by clinical interview. The interview considers 30 symptoms and each possible symptom is scored on a scale from 1–7. Apart from positive and negative symptomatology, the scale also considers the general psychopathology of the patient which pertains to somatic symptoms and indicators of depression and anxiety. This scale has been developed from the Brief Psychiatric Rating Scale (BPRS) referred to below.

- Brief Psychiatric Rating Scale (BPRS). Clinician and self-rated. Consists of 16–18 items. It enables clinicians to assess range of both psychotic and affective symptoms. A seven-point scale is used to score each item. The scale enables three scores to be generated for affective, negative and psychotic symptoms.

- Schedule for Assessment of Positive Symptoms (SAPS). Clinician-rated with use of interview. Will also take into account observed behaviours and feedback from nursing staff, relatives and the individual themselves. Assesses range of positive symptoms that occur in schizophrenia, namely formal thought disorder, hallucinations. Each item is scored on a scale of severity from 0–5.

- Schedule for Assessment of Negative Symptoms (SANS). Clinician-rated. Used in conjunction with the SAPS. As SAPS, it will consider observed behaviour, feedback from of the nursing team, relatives and individual themselves. Assesses range of negative symptoms that occur in schizophrenia including blunting of affect and poverty of speech. Each item is scored on a scale of severity from 0–5.

Rating scales: obsessive–compulsive disorder

Yale–Brown Obsessive Compulsive Scale is a clinician rated tool used to assess the severity of obsessive–compulsive symptoms. It is a ten-item scale of which the first five items pertain to obsessive symptoms and the latter five to compulsive symptoms. The severity of each symptom can also be indicated by an individual's response. The scale is also used to determine clinical improvement during treatment with appropriate psychotropic medication.

Rating scales: postnatal depression

Edinburgh Postnatal Depression Scale (EPDS) is a self-rated tool used to detect women at risk of postpartum depression. The scale consists of 10 items which cover a range of depressive symptoms including anhedonia, low mood and thoughts of self-harm. It considers how the woman has felt in the last seven days.

Rating scales: alcohol

There are a number of alcohol screening tests available to both the clinician and the individual. Perhaps the scale most familiar to us is the CAGE questionnaire as it is quick and straightforward to administer. The Closer look box outlines other tests commonly used in clinical practice.

 A CLOSER look...

Alcohol Screening Tests

- CAGE. The individual is asked the following four questions:

    – Have you ever felt that you should CUT DOWN on your drinking?

    – Have you ever felt ANNOYED by others criticising your drinking?

    – Have you ever felt GUILTY about the amount that you consume?

– Have you ever needed a drink first thing in the morning (an EYE-OPENER)?

An individual answering yes to >2 indicates a degree of alcohol dependence that would require further exploration.

- Alcohol Use Disorders Identification Test (AUDIT). Ten-item questionnaire used to detect harmful drinking behaviour and/or alcohol dependence. A score of 8 is indicative of harmful drinking behaviour whereas scores greater than 20 are a marker of alcohol dependence.

- Michigan Alcohol Screening Test (MAST). Accurate screening tool for alcohol dependence. Fairly time-consuming 22-item questionnaire. Considers lifetime drinking behaviour. A score of six or more is indicative of possible alcohol dependence and would require further exploration.

Rating scales: personality disorder

There are various scales used to screen for personality disorder, the majority of which prove to be vastly time-consuming and costly. If you are to remember any scales, it would be worth your while to remember the Minnesota Multiphasic Personality Inventory (MMPI) and the International Personality Disorder Examination (IPDE) for the purpose of the exam. Both are outlined in the Closer look box.

 A CLOSER look...

Personality disorder

- Minnesota Multiphasic Personality Inventory (MMPI). This is one of the most widely used assessment tools for personality disorder. It is self-rated, consisting of 567 statements with which the individual must respond with a TRUE/FALSE answer. It is vastly time-consuming and can take up to 2 hours to complete. The inventory is subdivided into various sub-scales that measure a degree of phenomenology including a depressive and hypomania (excitability) scale. It enables clinicians to identify both the structure of an individual's personality and associated psychopathology. Furthermore, it has a lie scale which enables clinicians to detect whether the patient is attempting to pick more favourable responses rather than those that are truly representative of them.

- International Personality Disorder Examination (IPDE). Compatible with ICD-10 and DSM-IV criteria. Semi-structured clinical interview that enables clinicians to reliably make a diagnosis of personality disorder. The examination considers six domains including work, affect, reality testing, self, impulse control and interpersonal relationships and relies on the patient's self-report and recall of symptoms over a lifetime.

Rating scales: eating disorder

The SCOFF questionnaire is a tool used by clinicians to detect the presence of a possible eating disorder in an individual. It consists of five questions and thus is quick and straightforward to administer. A positive response to two or more of the questions is indicative of a possible eating disorder. The questions are:

- Do you make yourself SICK when full?
- Are you worried that you have lost CONTROL of your eating?
- Have you lost more than ONE stone in weight over the last three months?
- Do you feel that you are FAT despite others saying to the contrary?
- Does FOOD dominate your life?

All the scales outlined above are commonly used in clinical practice. The MRCPsych exams also expect you to have a reasonable working knowledge of standardised assessment tools used in clinical research. Examples of those which commonly crop up time and time again are listed in the Closer look box.

 A CLOSER look...

Standardised assessment tools in clinical research

- Schedule for Assessment in Neuropsychiatry (SCAN). Development of the PSE. Consists of 28 sections. Uses CATEGO (an updated computerised diagnostic system) which enables clinicians to generate both ICD-10 and DSM-IV diagnoses.

Brief Psychiatric Rating Scale (BPRS). Mentioned briefly earlier in this chapter. Clinician- and self-rated. Consists of 16–18 items. It enables clinicians to assess the range of both psychotic and affective symptoms. A seven-point scale is used to score each item. The scale enables three scores to be generated for affective, negative and psychotic symptoms.

- Diagnostic Interview Schedule (DIS). Structured interview. Developed for the Epidemiological Catchment Area (ECA) Study. Can be administered by lay interviewers. Enables lifetime diagnoses.

- Structured Clinical Interview for Diagnosis (SCID). Enables DSM-IV diagnoses to be made. Administered by a clinician. Several versions exist including those for research. SCID-II version is available for personality disorders.

- Composite International Diagnostic Interview (CIDI). Developed for the World Health Organization (WHO). Can be administered by the lay interviewer and clinicians. Structured interview which enables ICD-10 and DSM-IV diagnoses to be made.

- General Health Questionnaire (GHQ). Screening tool used to ascertain minor psychiatric cases in a community, non-psychiatric population. It is self-rated. The scale is sensitive to short-term psychiatric disorders. Four versions exist: GHQ-12, GHQ-28, GHQ-30 and GHQ-60.

- Global Assessment of Functioning (GAQ). Considers individual's social, psychological and occupational functioning. Clinician-rated. Scale ranges from 0–100. Also constitutes the fifth axis of DSM-IV.

- Clinical Global Impression (CGI). Measure of global severity, seven-item scale. Assessors are asked to rate the severity of the patient's current illness in comparison to patients with similar diagnoses.

- Health of the Nation Outcome Scale (HONOS). Outcome measurement tool developed in response to government targets to improve health and social functioning of individuals with psychiatric disorders.

- Present State Examination (PSE). Used to identify psychiatric cases in a given population. Provides a measure of the individual's current mental state considering symptoms in the last four weeks. It enables clinicians to explore psychopathology and provide measures on a range of psychiatric conditions. It is however unsuitable in individuals with alcoholism, organic pathology and personality disorder. Development of a computer package CATEGO enables the information collated to be used to formulate a diagnosis.

Chapter 4

Basic psychology

Chapter 4
Basic psychology

Learning theory

Learning theories are an exam favourite. Easy marks can be gained here by revising some common themes, as outlined below.

 A CLOSER look...

Learning theories

Classical conditioning

- Also referred to in texts as 'Pavlovian conditioning'. A commonly used example to illustrate this theory is Pavlov's experiment on dogs. When food is presented to the dogs, the natural response is one of salivation. The salivation occurs *without condition*. The dog sees the food and it automatically makes them salivate. The food in this case is referred to as the 'unconditioned stimulus' and the salivation is referred to as the 'unconditioned response'.

Food ⟶ Salivation

Unconditioned stimulus   *Unconditioned response*

Pavlov later wished to consider whether introducing another stimulus (that would not naturally elicit salivation) alongside the food can cause the dogs to salivate even when the food is not presented.

In a process called conditioning, Pavlov introduced the sound of a bell each time the food was presented. The bell is referred to as the 'conditioned stimulus', i.e. the bell will cause the required salivatory response *on the condition* it is presented with the food.

Once the process of conditioning is complete, the dog will learn to salivate in response to presentation of the bell alone. The salivation elicited in response to the conditioned stimulus (the bell) is referred to as the conditioned response.

Bell   +   Food ⎯⎯⎯⎯⎯⎯⎯⎯⎯⟶ Salivation

Conditioned Stimulus   *Unconditioned stimulus Conditioned* response

A CLOSER look...

To guarantee the salivatory response, the experimenter must present the food (conditioned stimulus) *within 0.5 seconds* of the bell (conditioned stimulus) being rung, i.e. the closer together in time that the two stimuli are paired the more likely it is that the subject is able to make an association between the two and produce the desired response.

Further examples of pairing the UCS and CS.

a) *Simultaneous conditioning*. The UCS and CS are presented together, i.e. rather than 0.5 seconds apart.

b) *Forward conditioning*. This is the typical presentation whereby the CS is presented before the UCS, i.e. the bell is rung before the food is presented.

   Forward conditioning is further subdivided into two forms: Trace and Delay.

c) *Delay conditioning*. The CS is presented and the UCS follows some time later (a 'delay'). Using Pavlov's dog as an example, the bell is presented and then after a few seconds the food appears. The two stimuli co-exist. The shorter the delay between the two presentations, the stronger the association made by the subject.

d) *Trace conditioning*. The CS is presented and then removed. The food is then presented. The CS and UCS do not co-exist.

This process relies heavily on the subject's memory of the CS (the bell). If the subject (in this case the dog) is able to make an association between the bell and the food then conditioning has been successful.

e) *Backward conditioning*. Rather than the CS (bell) being presented first followed by the UCS (food), the food is presented first to the subject. Following which the bell is presented.

f) *Higher-order conditioning*. This process allows a second stimulus to be paired with the conditioned stimulus. For example, if a klaxon (a second stimulus) is paired with the bell, the conditioned response (the salivatory response) will be initiated by the sound of the klaxon alone.

Klaxon   +   Bell   +   Food ⟶ Salivation

The above example is referred to as second-order conditioning. If a neutral stimulus is simultaneously paired with the klaxon, this would be referred to as third-order conditioning.

Acquisition stage

When the subject is able to successfully make associations between the conditioned and unconditioned stimuli they are said to have achieved **acquisition**.

Extinction

This process occurs when the unconditioned stimulus is no longer paired with the conditioned stimulus, i.e. the food is no longer presented with the bell. As time progresses, the subject is no longer able to hold the association between the bell and food, subsequently losing the elicited conditioned response, i.e. salivation.

Spontaneous recovery

This refers to the process whereby presentation of the conditioned stimulus after extinction (i.e. after the association between CS and UCS is lost) will suddenly elicit a previous learned response, in this case salivation.

Learning processes and aetiological formulation of clinical problems

 A CLOSER look...

Learning processes

a) *Stimulus generalisation*. A stimulus that is similar to the conditioned stimulus can elicit the conditioned response. For example, a church bell and a hand bell can both equally cause the dog to salivate.

b) *Stimulus distinction*. The dog will not salivate in response to a doorbell. It is able to distinguish between the electronic sound of the doorbell and the authenticity of the hand bell. This highlights that the dog will only respond to a stimuli if it is presented in a particular form.

c) *Stimulus preparedness*. Describes the concept whereby certain individuals are more likely innately (be that through evolution) to respond to particular stimuli than others. Stimulus preparedness is used as an explanation as to why humans are more likely to fear spiders and snakes than other objects. This concept was put forward by Seligman.

d) *Incubation*. This contrasts with extinction. Please see definition above. Incubation refers to an increase in association between the CS and UCS despite disappearance of the UCS. For example, the conditioned stimulus, i.e the bell, need only be presented once before the association with the food is made. Repeated presentation of the bell without the food continues to elicit the salivatory response.

In the context of MRCPsych, a frequently used example is that of phobias. An individual learns to associate a spider with the feeling of fear even if they are only ever exposed to a spider once in their lifetime.

Operant conditioning

A process proposed by Skinner. This works on the principle that a subject modifies their behaviour depending on the consequences. Unlike classical conditioning, which works on the principle of the subject's reflex, i.e the dog's reflex of salivating in response to food is manipulated by introducing a neutral stimulus, operant conditioning makes use of the subject's surroundings or environment.

There are several concepts of operant conditioning with which you should familiarise yourself.

 A CLOSER look...

Learning theories

Operant conditioning

Reinforcement. Defined as a consequence which results in the subject increasing their behaviour. Reinforcement can be positive or negative but behaviour is always increased.

Positive reinforcement. A young girl is rewarded by her teacher with a gold star for every piece of homework she completes. The young girl knows that the more homework she completes the more stars she will receive so she ensures that she is diligent in her study. The reward (in this case the gold star) serves as the reinforcer to increase the desired behaviour of completing the homework.

Negative reinforcement. The same young girl has a gold star removed for every homework she fails to complete. The girl knows to avoid having stars deducted she needs to complete her homework. The removal of the aversive stimulus (in this case stars deducted) serves as the reinforcer to increase the desired behaviour of completing the homework.

Types of reinforcer: primary and secondary

Primary reinforcers are stimuli that innately 'reinforce' a behaviour and produce a desired response. Examples include food and warmth, i.e. the individual recognises this as an obvious reward and does not need to be conditioned to do so.

Secondary reinforcers, including money, are stimuli that are associated with primary reinforcers. Secondary reinforcers are associated with primary reinforcers through classical conditioning. An individual associates money with being able to buy food and warmth.

The impact of various reinforcement schedules

This works on the principle that the way the reinforcement is delivered can have an impact on the individual's response.

Reinforcers can be provided either continuously or intermittently. For example, every time a pupil scores an A grade, they are rewarded with a gold star, i.e. there is continuous reinforcement that good homework will receive a gold star. If a pupil is rewarded for a piece of homework on occasions only when the teacher feels they deserve a gold star, the pupil doesn't necessarily know when to expect a gold star and it seemingly occurs at random. This is referred to as intermittent reinforcement, as not every A grade is positively reinforced with a star.

Continuous reinforcement schedules are more likely to result in extinction. If a pupil suddenly stops receiving gold stars for every A grade, they may spend less time on their homework, receive poorer grades and adopt a 'what's the point of me trying to get the top grade if I don't get a star for it?' attitude.

In intermittent reinforcement schedules, extinction is less likely. The pupil knows that they will get a gold star for A-grade homework but that this could occur at any time. This pupil is more likely to continue performing well because they know 'at some point I will be rewarded for my homework'.

Intermittent schedules

There are different forms of intermittent schedules – ratio or interval – and these can be fixed or variable.

Ratio refers to the number of responses required before a reinforcer is produced. In fixed ratio schedules, a fixed predetermined number of responses are reinforced. In variable ratio schedules, any response can be reinforced.

Interval refers to the time interval that needs to lapse before a reinforcer is produced. In fixed interval schedules, each time a certain time period lapses a reinforcer is produced. In variable interval schedules, the reinforcement occurs at any given time.

A CLOSER look...

Learning theories

Intermittent reinforcement schedules

a) *Fixed ratio intermittent schedules.* A teacher rewards a pupil for every fourth piece of homework that receives an A grade.

b) *Variable ratio intermittent schedules.* A teacher rewards a pupil after their second A grade. A further reward is given after the pupil's sixth homework and then their ninth. The pupil is unaware of when the next reward (reinforcement) will occur.

c) *Fixed interval schedules.* A pupil is presented with a certificate after completing each year of study. The fixed interval in this case is one year.

d) *Variable interval schedules.* A pupil is presented with a certificate after the first year of study, then after the third year, then the fourth year and finally the sixth year. The time interval between each reinforcement varies.

The learning of desired behaviours is fastest when the individual is able to appreciate when their next reinforcement is due. Thus, fixed ratio reinforcement schedules allow for the quickest learning, whereas learning is slowest with a variable interval schedule.

Extinction (unlearning of a behaviour) is fastest with fixed ratio schedules. If an individual expects a reward for each desired behaviour carried out and suddenly stops receiving said reward, there is little incentive to carry out the behaviour so it is unlearned and the behaviour subsequently becomes extinct.

Variable interval schedules are most resistant to extinction as the individual has learnt that the reinforcement can occur at *any* time, therefore they will continue the behaviour until they receive (if at all) the expected reward.

Punishment

Unlike reinforcement which is used to increase a desired behaviour, punishment is used to reduce an undesired behaviour.

If we use the same schooling example as above:

At times, this young girl can spend hours doing her make-up in class rather than doing her work. The teacher continually gives her F grades and puts her in detention. The F grades and detention serve as a 'punishment' which reduces the undesired behaviour of applying make-up. The girl will subsequently concentrate on her studies to avoid the undesired consequence of poor grades and detention.

Punishment will always decrease a behaviour. Punishment can be positive or negative.

 A CLOSER look...

Punishment

a) *Positive punishment*. Describes adding an unpleasant stimulus after an undesired behaviour. By presenting the pupil with detention and poor grades, they are less likely to not perform well in their studies.

b) *Negative punishment*. Describes removing a pleasant stimulus after an undesired behaviour. By removing a gold star, the pupil is less likely to perform poorly at school.

Other forms of conditioning: escape and avoidance

Escape conditioning is a form of operant conditioning whereby an individual engages in a particular behaviour to terminate an aversive stimulus.

Example: an alarm sounds when an individual walks through a barrier at airport security. They then proceed to take off any metal items on their person which deactivates the alarm, i.e. terminates the unpleasant stimulus.

Avoidance conditioning is a form of operant conditioning whereby an individual prevents the unpleasant stimulus in the first place. This can be demonstrated in this example by the individual ensuring that they are not wearing anything that can sound the alarm in the first place, or removing this well in advance of the barrier if they are.

Clinical applications in behavioural treatments

 ### A CLOSER look...

Clinical applications

a) *Reciprocal inhibition.* This is based on the principle that two differing emotional states cannot co-exist. This can be demonstrated by the spider-phobic individual who has achieved a state of taught relaxation (an example being through meditation) who is then shown a spider. Reciprocal inhibition dictates that anxiety and relaxation cannot co-exist. The individual learns to displace the anxiety (which would be the usual response) related to the spider in favour of relaxation.

b) *Habituation.* Describes a graded approach to exposure. Using the example above, an individual may perhaps be:

- shown a picture of a spider first before

- shown a video of a moving spider

- made to hold a toy spider

- in the same room as a spider before progressing onto being able to hold one!

c) *Chaining.* Describes a series of stages that when completed in sequence result in an individual learning a complex task which would otherwise be difficult to learn.

An example could be teaching a young child to write their name. If the child's name is Sophie, rather than teach her how to write her name in full from the start (which would prove too difficult), instead this is broken down into manageable chunks that when interlinked will result in her being able to complete the task. At first, she learns that her name starts with the letter 'S'. When this stage is learnt and reinforced, she is able to move on to the letter 'O' and so on until the task is complete.

d) *Shaping*. This is different to chaining in that it allows 'successive approximations' to the intended learned task to be reinforced. So when an individual completes a task which has some resemblance to the final (expected) product they are still reinforced. A common example of shaping in practice is toilet training a young child.

f) *Flooding*. Used in the treatment of phobias. An individual is placed in the phobic situation with the presence of a therapist for a significant period of time. If we take the patient with the spider phobia, unlike habituation, flooding may require that the individual holds the spider without any graded exposure. The idea behind flooding is that it will evoke the usual anxiety response but that the individual will soon feel saturated with their fear response and that this will dissipate.

g) *Implosion*. Similar to flooding but rather than having the phobia present (*in vitro*), it is imagined (*in vivo*).

h) *Covert sensitisation*. Based on the principle that by imagining an unpleasant stimulus the individual is able to modify their behaviour. Example: a previously poorly controlled diabetic imagines the long-term complications of their condition every time they are tempted by a sugary treat. 'Imagining' these complications encourages them to avoid the chocolate bars and reach for a healthy snack instead.

i) *Overt sensitisation*. The opposite of covert sensitisation. Rather than imagining unpleasant stimuli, the individual is made to experience the unpleasant stimuli for themselves, which serves to modify the behaviour. An example of this is the use of disulfiram in the treatment of alcohol abuse. When an individual ingests alcohol while on disulfiram this results in unpleasant side effects which serve as the aversive stimulus.

Observational learning

Also referred to as modelling. Can be demonstrated by the influence that TV, media and live role models (parents) have on children in motivating them to mimic learned behaviours.

Basic principles of visual and auditory perception

Figure ground differentiation

Defined as the ability to distinguish an object from its environment.

Perceptual organisation: visual

The Closer look box describes the principles of how complex visual patterns are perceived and subsequently organised.

A CLOSER look...

Gestalt principles of perceptual organisation

- Continuity. Objects that are aligned together but otherwise distinct are seemingly grouped.

- Closure. Perceiving incomplete objects as a whole.

- Similarity. Images that look the same are automatically grouped together.

- Proximity. Objects perceived to be close together are grouped.

- Common fate. Objects moving together are grouped.

Information processing and attention: auditory

Broadbent's single channel (early selection) theory

- If several messages require processing, a filter will only select some of that information to be processed.

- The idea that we can't tend to more than one stimulus and only one piece of information can be processed at once.

Treisman's attenuation theory

- If an individual receives two messages, one of the messages is dampened down to focus on the other for information processing.

- If the other message is of relevance, however, the individual can switch their attention to the previously overlooked message.

Cherry's dichotic listening

- Presenting two different messages to both ears.

- Individuals are only able to attend to one message.

Deutsch–Norman theory

- All information is processed.

- Information is filtered later after processing is complete.

Memory

Three processes involved in the formation and subsequent access of memories.

- *Encoding*. Sensory input which leads to formation of the initial memory trace.

- *Storage*. Retention of the memory.

- *Retrieval*. Ability to access memory from storage.

Types of memory

- Sensory memory (visual memory lasts for 0.5 seconds, auditory memory lasts for 2 seconds)

- Short-term memory without the use of aides-memoires lasts 15–30 seconds. Capacity of 7 ± 2 distinct items. Can be increased by chunking.

- Long-term memory has unlimited capacity.

A CLOSER look...

Chunking

- Allows individuals to combine several items into larger pieces of information which are more easily recalled by a user.

- An example of this is remembering a telephone number. Individuals will normally not remember each number independently if given a nine-digit number.

0 1 2 3 4 567890

But by chunking and pairing digits to one another, a nine-digit number becomes much easier to manage and subsequently recall.

01-23-45-67-89-0

Types of long-term memory

Long-term memory can be further subdivided into declarative and non-declarative memory.

- Semantic and episodic memory are examples of declarative (explicit) memory.

- Procedural memory is an example of non-declarative (implicit) memory.

 A CLOSER look...

Long-term memory

- *Semantic memory*. Refers to general knowledge memory.

- *Episodic memory*. Memories related to the self.

- *Flashbulb memory*. Type of episodic memory where individuals are able to specifically recall what they were doing at times of significant events.

- *Procedural memory*. Memory for knowing how to perform a particular skill.

Forgetting

Several theories exist on how we forget previously learned information. Interference with any of the three processes involved in memory formation – encoding, storage and retrieval – can result in forgetting.

Decay (disuse) theory

- Suggests without continued use or rehearsal, memories fade over time.

Interference theory

- Subdivided into two types: proactive and retroactive interference.
- Proactive interference describes difficulty in learning new information due to the presence of older material.
- Retroactive interference describes difficulty in recalling old material due to learning of new material.

Displacement theory

- Old material is replaced by new material. New material displaces previously learnt items.

Failure of retrieval

- Difficult to recall items due to lack of cues. *Example*: a postgraduate student is able to recall their university days and associated happiness each time they play a song that would previously be on repeat at the Union bar.

Memory disorders

Anterograde amnesia	Difficulty in forming new memories.
	Hence information cannot be moved from short-term to long-term memory.
	Damage to hippocampus typically presents with this.
Retrograde amnesia	Difficulty in recalling older memories.
	Hence information cannot be moved from long-term to short-term memory.

Head trauma typically presents with this pattern of amnesia with failure to recall memories prior to the injury.

Korsakoff's syndrome	Severe anterograde and retrograde amnesia.
	Working memory and implicit (procedural) memory spared.
	Associated with chronic alcohol abuse.
Dissociative fugue	Associated period of wandering.
	Sudden loss of episodic memory and personal identity.
	Transient with recovery of memory.

Personality

Derivation of nomothetic and idiographic theories

Nomothetic	The idea that personalities can be classified and traits can be shared by individuals.
Idiographic	The idea that personalities are unique and distinct.

Several theories on personality exist, some of the common proponents of which are listed below. These tend to make for easy mark scoring in multiple choice questions and extended matched items.

A CLOSER look...

Personality theories.

- Costa's Big 5: Agreeablenss, Conscientousness, Neuroticism, Extraversion, Openess (ACNE-O)

- Eysenck: Three-dimensional traits with lie scale.

    – Neuroticism–stability

    – Extraversion–introversion

    – Psychoticism.

- Kelly's Personal Construct Theory proposes that individuals relate to the world through hypothetical constructs.

- Allport's Trait Theory. Identified three traits: central, cardinal and secondary.

- Cattell distinguished between source and surface traits. Identified 16 source traits that are fundamental to personality.

Use of inventories and rating scales

Minnesota and Multiphasic Inventory (MMPI) and International Personality Disorder Examination (IPDE) have previously been mentioned in Chapter 3, Diagnostic tools and rating scales chapter. These are both examples of objective tests for personality. Personality can also be rated by means of projective testing. Projective tests, unlike objective tests, do not use a universal standard with which to compare the individual.

 A CLOSER look...

Projective tests

- Rorschach's inkblot test

- Sentence completion

- Draw a person

- Thematic apperception test

Motivation

Defined as the process that initiates and maintains goal-directed behaviours. Theories on motivation are often subdivided into intrinsic and extrinsic theories.

Extrinsic theories

- External factors motivate individuals, e.g. standing to gain reward from their behaviour.

Homeostatic theory

- Imbalance of psychological and physiological equilibrium creates a need.

  Example: a diabetic becomes drowsy due to a drop in blood sugars. This disturbs a physiological equilibrium. This creates a need for the individual to drink a sugary drink. This drives and motivates them to locate a sugary drink. Once they consume the drink the balance in blood sugars is restored.

Intrinsic theory

- Internal factors motivate individuals.

  Example: A woman is tired after a long day at work and returns home where she lives alone. One of her friends rings her and asks her to come round for dinner. The woman is motivated (despite her tiredness) at being able to have some company and so goes round. Her comfort-seeking behaviour serves as the motivation factor.

Maslow's hierarchy of needs

- Proposed a theory on human motivation.

- Identifies two types of needs: D and B.

- Lower needs (D) to be satisfied before entertaining higher needs (B).

- Deficiency (D) needs are physiological needs, safety and security, love and belongingness and self-worth (esteem) needs.

- Being (B) or growth needs are aesthetic and self-actualisation needs.

Emotion

Emotion can be characterised by:

- the subjective experience (what the patient *feels*)

- cognition (what the patient *thinks* about the emotion)

- physiological response (how does the *body behave*)

- subsequent behaviour (how the *individual responds* to the emotion).

Several theories exist with regard to emotion. Proponents of these theories are commonly cited in the Membership exams, namely Cannon–Bard, James–Lange, Schachter and Singer and Lazarus.

A CLOSER look...

Theories of emotion

- **James–Lange**. Physiological changes occur first in response to a stimulus. This response feeds back to the cortex and the individual is able to perceive emotion.

- **Cannon–Bard**. In response to a stimulus, the cortex (via the thalamus) enables the interpretation of the emotion. Simultaneously, the hypothalamus leads to physiological changes.

- **Schachter and Singer's Labelling Theory**. In response to a stimulus, bodily arousal and a physiological response occurs. The individual will then interpret the emotion and label it as positive or negative depending on situational cues.

  Example: A core trainee attends an interview. He notices his heart is racing. He interprets this as the emotion of fear because he is at an interview.

- **Lazarus' Cognitive Appraisal**. This proposes that emotions are secondary to how we 'appraise' or think about a situation.

  Example: The core trainee above thinks 'I'm going for an interview. I don't think they will give me a job.' He subsequently feels nervous and as a result his heart races and he begins to feel sweaty.

Chapter 5

Human development

Chapter 5
Human development

Attachment theory

John Bowlby is the proponent of attachment theory.

Phases of attachment

Pre-attachment process | 0–3 months
Orientation to mothers

Indiscriminate attachment | 3–6 months
Can form attachments to several individuals or strangers. Not necessarily primary caregiver.

Discriminate attachment | 6–24 months
Attachment becomes less general and more clear-cut as the child identifies preferential attachment figures.

 A CLOSER look...

Milestones of attachment

- Stranger anxiety typically occurs between 6 and 12 months.

- Attachment behaviour typically occurs between ages of 12 and 18 months.

Other proponents of attachment

Ainsworth

Ainsworth identified four types of attachment behaviour – secure, anxious-avoidant, anxious-resistant and disorganised. The Closer look box describes the Strange Situation Experiment developed by Ainsworth and used to identify these attachment subtypes.

 A CLOSER look...

Ainsworth's strange situation experiment

Stage 1 Mother and Child in room

Stage 2 Joined by stranger

Stage 3 Mother leaves; child is left with stranger   SEPARATION

Stage 4 Mother comes back; stranger leaves   REUNION

Stage 5 Mother leaves; child is left alone   SEPARATION

Stage 6 Stranger returns and attempts to comfort child

Stage 7 Mother returns; stranger leaves   REUNION

NB Ainsworth identified two separation and two reunion episodes between mother and child.

Types of attachment behaviour

Anxious-avoidant (Type A)   Fifteen per cent of infants classified as this subtype.

Environment-dependent.

No emotion when separated or reunited with mother

Shows distress when left alone

Can be easily comforted by strangers

Secure (Type B)	Seventy per cent of infants classified as this subtype
	Happy when present with mother
	Shows distress when separated from mother and immediately seeks comfort on her return
	Stranger unsuccessful in comforting child
Anxious-resistant (Type C)	Fifteen per cent classified into this subtype
	Highly distressed when separated from mother but is not successfully comforted on her return
	Resists stranger's attempt to comfort
Disorganised (Type D)	Fearful of mother
	Attempts to seek comfort from mother but this in itself induces fear

Main's adult attachment behaviour

Main developed an attachment interview used on adults to enable the interviewer to predict their attachment behaviour in childhood. The interviewer focuses on how the adult is able to recall childhood memories.

Four subtypes exist: autonomous, dismissing, entangled and disorganised.

 A CLOSER look...

Adult attachment

- **Dismissing**. Adults minimise their childhood experiences upon recollection. They don't 'dress it up'. Predicts anxious-avoidant (Type A) childhood attachment.

- **Secure autonomous**. Able to talk at length and without distress about both positive and negative childhood experiences. Predicts secure (Type B) childhood attachment.

- **Entangled**. Very emotional and lengthy account of their childhood. Predicts anxious-resistant (Type C) childhood attachment.

- **Disorganised**. As the title suggests, the adult provides a very disorganised account of their childhood. Predicts disorganised (Type D) childhood attachment.

Mahler's separation individuation theory

This theory highlights the stages through which a child passes in being able to develop a sense of identity distinct from the mother.

It consists of three phases:

- **Normal autism:** 0–2 months. Spends majority of time sleeping.

- **Symbiosis:** 2–5 months. Views mother and self as one.

- **Separation individuation phase:** 5 months–5 years.

The separation individuation phase is further subdivided into:

- **Differentiation**. Able to see a difference between mother and self.

- **Practicing**. Begins to explore environment.

- **Rapprochment**. Continues to explore environment but seeks reassurance from mother upon return.

- **Object constancy**. Appreciates that self and mother are distinct. Acknowledges that even if mother is not visible she is not gone forever.

Cognitive development

Piaget is the main proponent of this theory. It consists of four stages:

- Sensorimotor

- Pre-operational

- Concrete operational

- Formal operational.

A CLOSER look...

Piaget's cognitive development

- Sensorimotor, 0–2 years:
  - Imitative play
  - Symbolism
  - Self-recognition
  - Object permanence.

- Preoperational, 2–7 years:
  - Animism
  - Transductive reasoning
  - Egocentric thinking. Only able to see things from their point of view. 'The Mountain Experiment' demonstrates this well
  - Lack of conservation.

- Concrete operational, 7–11 years:
  - Conservation achieved.

    Example: able to appreciate that when 100mls water is transferred from a short flask into a tall, slim flask the taller flask still holds the same volume of water, despite looking as though it should hold more.

- Formal operational, 11 years +
  - Abstract thinking
  - Able to carry out mental operations
  - Thirty per cent of adults do not reach this stage

Language development

0–12 months	Cooing (6 weeks)
	Babbling (9 months)
12–18 months	One word
	Holophrases where one word is representative of a whole sentence
18–30 months	Telegraphic speech. Pairing words of meaning
	Vocabulary of >240 words
30 months	Early appreciation of grammar and sentence form
48 months	Correct use of grammar
60 months	Adult speech

Motor development

3 months	Able to hold head up
6 months	Able to sit up
	Pincer grip
	Picking up objects
12 months	Able to stand alone briefly
18–24 months	Walks independently
	Able to walk up and down stairs with handrails
	Able to use a spoon
	Can build tower three–four cubes high
24 months	Able to run
	Can build tower six cubes high
36 months	Able to walk up and down stairs independently
	Can build tower of nine cubes
48 months	Able to skip

Development in drawing skills

3 years	Able to draw a circle
4 years	Able to draw a 'plus' sign
4.5 years	Able to draw a square
5 years	Able to draw a triangle
7 years	Able to draw a rhomboid shape

Fear development

0–6 months	Loud noises
	Falling
6–12 months	Stranger anxiety
	Heights
12 months	Stranger anxiety
	Separation anxiety
24–36 months	The dark
	Animals
5–8 years	Imaginary animals: monsters
9–12 years	Fear of world disasters and injuries
Adolescence	Fear of peers and social pressures

Moral development

Kohlberg is the main proponent of moral development.

There are three levels identified which in turn are further subdivided into two phases.

Level 1	Preconventional morality
Level 2	Conventional morality
Level 3	Postconventional morality

A CLOSER look...

Kohlberg's moral development

Level 1 Preconventional morality

Stage 1   Obeying of rules to avoid punishment. Obedience/ punishment-orientated.

Stage 2   Obeying of rules to receive reward

Level 2 Conventional morality

Stage 3   Good boy/good girl orientation. Behaviour in order to gain approval from others.

Stage 4   Obeys authority and social ruling.

Level 3 Postconventional morality

Stage 5   Behaviour guided by social contract and democracy.

Stage 6   Behaviour guided by universal, self-defined principles.

Erikson's psychosocial development

0–18 months	Trust vs mistrust
18–36 months	Autonomy vs shame
3–6 years	Initiative vs guilt
6–11 years	Industry vs inferiority
Adolescence	Identity vs role confusion
Young adult	Intimacy vs isolation
Adulthood	Generativity vs stagnation
Old age	Ego integrity vs despair

Psychosexual development

Proposed by Freud. Consists of five stages: oral, anal, phallic, lateny and genital.

0–18 months	Oral stage	Mouth is the focus of libido gratification.
		Using the mouth to explore their environment, e.g. breastfeeding, sucking, putting objects in mouth.
		Fixation at this stage is thought to explain addiction behaviours such as smoking.
18–36 months	Anal stage	The anus becomes the erogenous zone.
		Example: toilet training
		Fixation at this stage may lead to obsessive personality (anal retention) or disorganisation (anal expulsion)
3–5 years	Phallic stage	Genitals become erogenous zone.
		Oedipus and Electra complex.
		Oedipus complex or 'castration anxiety' in boys, where boys compete with father for mother's attention and love.
		Electra complex or 'penis envy' where girls resent mother for absence of penis. Wanting to bear father's child.
		Successfully achieving the phallic stage results in the boy/girl identifying with the same-sex parent.

5 years–puberty	Latent stage	Gratification instincts lay 'latent'. Socialisation. Early genital sexual development.
Puberty>	Genital stage	Genital exploration

Chapter 6

Social psychology

Chapter 6
Social psychology

Attitudes

Attitudes comprise three basic components – affective, behavioural and cognitive, ABC – and are defined as an individual's evaluation and response to a certain stimulus.

A CLOSER look...

Attitude – remember ABC

- Affective: 'Feelings'

  How the individual feels about a given situation.

- Behavioural: 'Action'

  How the individual responds to a given situation.

- Cognitive: 'Thoughts'

  What the individual thinks about a given situation.

Measurement of attitude

Attitudes can be measured using a number of methods:

- Direct observation
- Self-report
- Interviews

- Use of scales: Thurstone, Osgood Semantic Differential and Likert.

A criticism of the direct observation method suggests that the observed behaviour of an individual is not necessarily a reflection of their attitude.

There is also a concern that encouraging self-reporting may encourage a social desirability bias as subjects give what they perceive to be more favourable responses.

A CLOSER look...

Likert

- Five-point scale
- Assesses subject's level of agreement/disagreement to a number of statements.

Example:

The MRCPsych Paper 1 Exam is challenging.

Strongly agree	Agree	Neither agree nor disagree	Disagree	Strongly disagree
5	4	3	2	1

A CLOSER look...

The Thurstone scale

- More time-consuming than the Likert!
- A number of statements with a common theme are presented to an independent judging panel who score them using an 11-point response scale (from 1 being very negative to 11 very positive).
- The average scores for each statement are obtained and a numerical value assigned to each.
- A selection of sample statements are taken and presented to an individual.

A CLOSER look...

The communicator

- Expert in their field and credible
- Likeable
- Attractive
- Similarity; audience able to identify with communicator
- Proximity to audience
- Genuine in delivery of message
- Motivated

The audience

- Recipients with low self-esteem are more likely to be receptive to a simpler message.
- Recipients with high self-esteem are more likely to be receptive to a more complex message.
- Levels of intelligence are important factors to bear in mind, as detailed below.
- Increased vulnerability in the recipient makes persuasion more successful.

The message

- Element of fear. In individuals with low anxiety levels this can prove effective. However, it can prove counterproductive if the recipients are highly anxious.
- An explicit message and presenting one-sided arguments is more persuasive in the less intelligent.
- An implicit message and presenting two-sided arguments is more successful in the more intelligent.

Self-psychology

Familiarise yourselves with these simple definitions. These make for easy point-scoring should they crop up as an EMI.

Self concept	Multifaceted. Incorporates how an individual views themself and how they perceive others to view them.
Self-consciousness	Awareness of self as distinct from its environment and objects within it.
Self-esteem	Individual's sense of self-worth.
Ideal self	What an individual would like to be.
Self-image	How an individual describes themselves both in terms of physical characteristics, disposition and their role in society.
Self recognition	Can be demonstrated with the 'rouge test'. This is a test conducted in front of a mirror whereby a red dot is unknowingly placed on a child's forehead. If the child (through exploration in front of the mirror) is able to identify that the 'rouge' spot is a part of them they will have successfully achieved 'self-recognition'. This typically occurs between the ages of 18 and 20 months.

Interpersonal issues

Attribution theory

Attribution is a cognitive process which allows us to interpret the behaviour of ourselves and others and to consider causes for observed behaviours.

Kelley's covariation model of attribution considered three components useful in determining attribution: consistency, consensus and distinctiveness.

A CLOSER look...

Attribution theory

Example: Mrs Y was observed by her husband (Mr Y) to not turn up to an event held by Mr and Mrs Z. Mr Y wants to consider the causes (attributional factors) for this.

Consistency: Does Mrs Y always not turn up to Mr and Mrs Z's events?

Consensus: Do all the other neighbours also not turn up to Mr and Mrs Z's events?

Distinctiveness: Is it only Mr and Mrs Z's event that she doesn't turn up to or does she avoid events held by all neighbours?

Using the above Mr Y could make several inferences:

- If consistency is high, he could attribute her behaviour to be due to not liking Mr and Mrs Z's event.

- If consensus is low, he could attribute her behaviour to be specific to her, i.e. relating it to dispositional/personality issues.

Other theories of attribution were proposed by Weiner and Heider. Weiner considered a three-dimensional model of attribution. This theory relates specifically to achievement. Consider the student who studies for an exam in the example below.

A CLOSER look...

Weiner's three-dimensional model

- Stability (stable and unstable)

- Locus of control (internal and external)

- Controllability (controllable and uncontrollable)

A student fails an exam. If we consider that this failure is stable, with internal locus and is controllable, we can infer that:

The student always fails exams (stable behaviour), that it is related to the individual not being a fan of studying (internal) and that it is within the individual's control to study harder (controllable).

Heider proposed an early theory of attribution. He distinguished internal (dispositional) from external (situational) causality. An internal causality suggests an individual is directly responsible for the outcome, whereas an external causality suggests that an outside agent is responsible.

We can use the same example as above to illustrate this point: X fails an exam and attributes this to the exam being unfair (situational/external causality). However, when X's friend fails an exam he attributes this to his friend not studying hard enough (dispositional/internal).

Attributional biases

Interpretations of observed behaviours (attribution) can be subject to bias.

Fundamental attribution error	When observing other people's behaviours particularly if the observed behaviour is negative, we are likely to infer causality to dispositional factors rather than situational factors.
Self-serving bias	Attributing one's own failures to be due to situational/external factors and attributing success to dispositional/internal causality.

Leadership

The characteristics demonstrated by a leader are dependent on several factors, including:

- Characteristics of the group.

- The requirements of the task.

Lewin identified three different leadership styles – laissez-faire, autocratic, democratic – and the effects this has on the group. He also identified how the leader interacts with the group, how the groups interact with their leader and how this impacts on their ability to complete a task. It also explores the behaviour of the group in the absence of the leader. This is outlined in more detail in the Closer look box.

A CLOSER look...

Leadership

- Laissez-faire refers to a relaxed, hands-off approach to leading. Such leadership style proves effective in individuals who are highly skilled and require little guidance. In situations where group members are less skilled and not used to having to 'fend for themselves', this style of leadership can prove troublesome. Group members may stray from the task at hand if they are not guided in completing it.

- Autocratic describes an aggressive form of leadership whereby the leader is responsible for all decision-making with very minimal input from group members. This method can be useful in the completion of highly complex tasks with deadlines that need to be met where guidance by a leader who can delegate tasks efficiently is required. This increases the likelihood of task completion. The disadvantages of such a style are that an overly autocratic leader can risk alienating group members. Members may also resent the leader for not taking into account views of the group. As a result in the absence of the leader, members are observed to abandon the task.

- Democratic describes a supportive approach to leadership where contribution by group members is actively encouraged. Tasks are completed to time and creatively because group members feel involved and appreciated. This style of leadership typically boosts team morale. In the absence of a leader, individuals are shown to continue with the task at hand.

Social influence and power

Social power describes the process whereby individuals are able to exert influence on others. French and Raven identified five types of social power: authority, coercion, expertise, referential and reward.

 A CLOSER look...

French and Raven's social power

- Authority suggests that status/role of an individual may bear some influence over others.

- Coercion describes how the use of punishment may bear influence on others.

- Expertise applies if an individual is deemed an expert or knowledgeable in their field.

- Referential describes how an individual associated with other potentially influencial people. Liked/admired by others.

- Rewarding others may be influential.

Obedience

Obedience describes an individual's compliance to an instruction from authority. This was famously demonstrated in Stanley Milgram's experiments where subjects were asked to deliver electric shocks to their victims.

 A CLOSER look...

Stanley Milgram obedience experiments

- Subjects adopted the role of 'teacher' and were instructed by white-coated professionals (authority) to 'teach' various tasks to their 'victims'.

- The victims were then asked a series of questions based on common themes they had learnt from their teacher.

- Unbeknownst to the teacher, the 'victim' was in fact an actor.

- For each response the victim got wrong the white-coated professional instructed the subjects to deliver an electric shock. The subjects were led to believe that the electric shocks were real when in fact they were not.

- The actor (the victim) would shriek each time a shock was delivered.

- For every incorrect response, an electric shock of increased charge was delivered by the teacher upon instruction by the white-coated professional.

The experiment highlights the impact that a perceived authority figure can have on an individual, even in a situation where they perceive wrongdoing, namely delivering a potentially lethal electric shock to an unknown victim.

Influence operating in small and large groups or crowds

Conformity describes the process whereby an individual is observed to bow down to the pressure of others in a group situation. Individuals tend to demonstrate conformity to avoid the risk of being ousted or rejected from a group.

Conformity increases the more members there are in the group and the more influential individual group members are.

Other factors that determine conformity include:

- Intelligence

- Self-reliance

- Expressiveness.

Individuals who were of high intelligence, self-reliant and expressive were less likely to bow down to the pressures of the group and conform.

Group processes

A CLOSER look...

Group processes

- **Groupthink** describes the process whereby group members lean towards unanimity (everyone coming to the same agreement) even if this is at the risk of suppressing their own opinions.

  Groupthink typically occurs in a high-pressured task where individuals are rushed to complete it. An autocratic (aggressive) leader can also encourage groupthink as members are led into a decision that perhaps they would not ordinarily make.

- In **group polarisation** individuals make their own individual decisions, but then decide on the same matter as a group. The decision tends to be more extreme.

- **Risky shift**. Fairly self-explanatory. The group decision is more 'risky' than what an individual would perhaps make on their own.

- **Deindividuation** describes how the whole of the group is more important than its individual members.

- **Group membership**, namely ingroup and outgroup.

- **Ingroup** is defined as any group with which an individual is able to identify. This group is perceived as heterogenous: 'everyone's different'.

- **Outgroup** is defined as a group that an individual is not able to identify with when coming into contact with them. This group is perceived as homeogenous: 'they're all the same'.

Intergroup behaviour

Membership to particular groups can subject individuals to prejudice, stereotyping and subsequently intergroup hostility.

Prejudice is defined as an attitude towards individuals based on their membership of a particular group. It can be used to describe positive, negative and impartial attitudes. There are a number of theories for prejudice, as demonstrated in the Closer look box.

Sterotyping describes a cognitive process whereby individuals harbour over-generalised beliefs about members of particular groups. It involves a form of social categorisation whereby we infer preconceived ideas of others.

A CLOSER look...

Theories of prejudice

- **Realistic conflict theory**. Suggests that when different groups are required to compete with one another for the same resources it creates intergroup hostility.

- **Frustration aggression theory** (scapegoating). Describes how individuals in the same group at times of difficulty and/ or relative deprivation displace their frustration and attack outgroup targets.

- **Adorno's authoritarian personality theory**. Most common in individuals who have had a difficult, harsh upbringing who may in turn project their own difficulties onto others.

  Social identity. Identification with their own group can lead to prejudice against any 'outgroups'.

Many have proposed theories on ways to reduce prejudice and intergroup hostility. Allport proposed the contact hypothesis. He proposed that prejudice could be reduced by putting two distinct groups into contact with one another and giving them an opportunity to correct their stereotypes/preconceptions of the 'outgroup' and enabling them to work together in pursuit of a common goal.

Aggression

Aggression is defined as behaviour with intent to harm others. It can be sub-categorised further, as discussed in the Closer look box.

A CLOSER look...

Aggression

- **Covert aggression**. Subtle. Includes methods such as telling lies.

- **Overt aggression**. More blatant. Can be observed.

- **Hostile aggression**. Is for the purpose of hurting an individual.

- **Pathological aggression**. This is being aggressive for the sake of it, i.e unlike hostile aggression, it is not necessarily to hurt someone.

- **Instrumental aggression**. This is aggression for in order to attain something i.e. sense of purpose.

- **Positive aggression** can be best represented in acts such as self-defence where aggression is used for the sole purpose of protection.

Theories of aggression

Several theories have been proposed as explanations for aggression. These include the social learning theory, operant conditioning, frustration–aggression hypothesis, psychoanalysis and ethnology. There is also a suggestion that television and the media may have some influence. Family and social backgrounds are also thought to play a part.

A CLOSER look...

Theories of aggression

- **Ethnology**. This theory proposes that aggression is inborn. It states that in situations in which we are trapped and faced with an unfamiliar threat the natural response would be to reciprocate aggression.

- **Operant conditioning**. This can best be demonstrated in the example of a bull terrier who is rewarded by his owner for acts of aggression against an unsuspecting stuffed toy. Each time the dog carries out an aggressive act he is given a dog treat. The dog treat works as a positive reinforcement for continued acts of aggression.

- **Social learning theory**. This is best demonstrated by Bandura's Bobo Doll Experiment. This is based on the theory that aggression is learnt through observational learning (modelling). In this experiment, when a child is observed by other children to be aggressive towards a target (in this case, a doll) and seemingly rewarded for such behaviour, the children are observed to 'model' (mimic) this aggression.

- **Dollard's frustration–aggression theory**. This proposes the idea that times of increased frustration can lead to aggressive acts. When an unsuspecting target is the focus of the aggression, this is called scapegoating. This theory suggests that where there is frustration there is always aggression and where there is aggression there is always frustration – one does not exist without the other.

- Unlike Dollard's theory, **Berkowitz's aggressive cue theory** proposes that frustration does not necessarily lead to aggression, but that instead it makes an individual more likely to respond aggressively in the presence of environmental cues.

Television and media influences

Based on the principle of modelling. This suggests that through observation of aggressive acts via the media (through television or computer games, for example), individuals are encouraged to mimic learned behaviours.

Theory of interpersonal attraction

Certain factors are thought to influence interpersonal attraction and friendship:

- Similarity

- Familiarity

- Proximity

- Physical attractiveness

- Exposure (namely reciprocal self-disclosure)

- Reciprocal liking

- Complementarity (more important for sustaining the relationship in long term).

These hold true for individuals seeking support from others, be it in the short term, through friendship formation or long-term companionship.

Parenting

 A CLOSER look...

Parenting

- **Permissive**. Make few demands of their children. Exert little control. Are very nurturing. Low expectations of their children. Act as a friend more than a parent. Inadequate interpersonal communication.

- **Neglectful**. Make few demands of their children. Have little control. Are not nurturing. Detached from their children's life and do not meet basic needs. Poor communication.

- **Authoritarian**. Place high demands on their children. Strict rules which children are expected to follow without question. Very controlling. Poor nurturance. Have high expectations of their children. Poor communication.

- **Authoritative**. Place demands on their children that are appropriate. More democratic. Discipline children in a supportive manner. Good level of control. Nurturing. Have expectations for their children which are age appropriate. Good level of communication.

Altruism

Altruism is defined as a helping behaviour that is motivated by putting the interests of others before one's own. Different types of helping behaviours make for a simple MCQ/EMI so are worth remembering.

 A CLOSER look...

Helping behaviours

- **Bystander effect/apathy** (Genovese effect). A phenomenon whereby in an emergency situation where an individual requires help, intervention is less likely the more bystanders there are observing.

- **Diffusion of responsibility** describes the phenomenon whereby individuals are less likely to take responsibility for an action if others are present. 'Why do I have to help? Why doesn't someone else?'

- **Dissolution of responsibility**. 'I'm sure someone else will have helped.'

- **Pluralistic ignorance** describes a phenomenon where an individual will 'follow the crowd' because they believe that is what others expect from them in this situation. If we use the example of an individual taking up smoking. In a group of fellow smokers, the individual will look at others and it would seem that others are 'enjoying' smoking, so the individual continues and gives the impression that he is similarly enjoying it. The individual may be unaware that others are suppressing similar feelings of displeasure but because no-one admits that they believe that others are enjoying smoking.

- **Social exchange theory** works on the principle that individuals engage in helping behaviours with the idea that 'the favour will be returned' at some point.

Social science and sociocultural psychiatry

Social class and socio-economic status play an important role, particularly when considering the epidemiology of psychiatric disorders and subsequent healthcare delivery. Social class is defined as a means of categorising a group of individuals based on education, occupation and income.

A CLOSER look...

Social class

- Social class I: Professional
- Social class II: Intermediate
- Social class III: Skilled
- Social class IV: Semi-skilled
- Social class V: Unskilled
- Social class O: Unemployed

Social class has been implicated as contributing to the incidence and prevalence of psychiatric disorders. It is proposed that the environmental stresses that lower classes are subjected compared with their higher-class counterparts plays a considerable role.

Psychiatric disorders are more common in individuals in lower social classes. Exceptions to this pattern are bipolar affective disorder and eating disorders, which are more prevalent in the higher classes. Individuals in lower classes are more likely to be admitted to inpatient facilities and to be subjected to more aggressive therapies, e.g. ECT.

In 1980, Goldberg and Huxley proposed a psychiatric healthcare model that attempts to identify 'filters' through which individuals in the community pass in order to access psychiatric care. How readily they pass through this framework is dependent on factors including socio-economic status (SES).

A CLOSER look...

Goldberg and Huxley's (1980) filter model of psychiatric healthcare

Filter 1: Individual recognises symptoms which prompt help-seeking behaviour.

Filter 2: GP diagnoses mental health disorder.

Filter 3: Referral to specialist services.

Filter 4: Admission to specialist inpatient unit.

The sociology of residential institutions

With the introduction of new psychotropic medications and with an increasing shift towards community psychiatric treatments, the process of deinstitutionalisation began as a means of avoiding unnecessary admissions to inpatient facilities and providing delivery of services in the community.

It is still important to have an awareness of total institutions for the exam. Goffman is commonly cited in psychiatric text for his work on asylums. He studied the process of institutionalisation, specifically considering the role of the patient.

A CLOSER look...

Goffman's total institutions

- **Total institution**. Examples include traditional asylums which see individuals isolated from the outside world and all aspects of life: work, home life and play all occur under one roof.

- **Mortification process**. Series of processes that see an individual move from the outside world to being an inhabitant of the total institution.

- **Betrayal funnel** describes how individuals pass from the care of their relatives to the care of the health professional. There is a sense that the patient has been 'betrayed' by their own family and resents them for 'handing them over'.

- **Role stripping**. Upon admission to the asylum, the individual is 'stripped' of normal social roles and their previous identity and submits to their new patient role.

- **Binary management** describes how the worlds of the staff and residents are viewed as being very much distinct both socially and culturally.

- **Batch living** describes how individuals are seen as a group governed by rules and regulations, all are treated alike.

Chapter 7

Ethics

Chapter 7
Ethics

Basic ethics

Deontology and teleology are two terms commonly used when referring to ethical principles in medical practice.

A CLOSER look...

Deontology

- 'Duty-based' approach.

- Originates from the Greek word *deon* meaning 'duty'.

- Rules and obligations determine action.

- Concerned with what individuals do and not the consequence of the action.

- Commonly associated terms: moral absolutism, prima facie, duty proper.

- Prima facie.

Teleology

- 'Utilitarian-based' approach.

- Originates from the Greek word *teleon* meaning 'purpose'.

- Action determined by the 'greatest good for the greatest number'.

- Concerned with the consequences of action.

- Commonly associated terms: Utilitarianism, consequentialism.

- Utilitarianism/consequentialism – the correct action is the one with the most favourable outcome.

Common names in ethics

It is worthwhile spending some time to familiarise yourself with these.

Kant	'Moral philosophy'
Ross	'Prima facie' obligations.
Beauchamp and Childress	The four principles of biomedical ethics.

 A CLOSER look...

Beauchamp and Childress

- **Autonomy**. Respecting an individual's right to make their own choice.

- **Beneficience**. Right to 'do good'.

- **Non-maleficence**. 'To do no harm'.

- **Justice**. Equally distributing resources. To act fairly.

 A CLOSER look...

William David Ross

- Moral realist.

- Seven prima facie obligations, including fidelity, gratitude, reparation.

- Determine what an individual 'ought' to do in any given ethical dilemma.

Other ethical theories

Virtue theory	Focuses on the individual and their characteristics, i.e. not duty-based.
	Identifies desirable moral and intellectual qualities that individuals should aspire towards to lead a good life.
Pragmatic theory	Goal-oriented. Achieving success with little regard as to how this is achieved.
Humanistic ethics	Guided by 'what's best for society'.

Research ethics

Studies to be familiar with include Tuskegee Syphilis Study, Nuremberg Trials and Helsinki and Geneva Declarations. They have been known to pop up in the odd MCQ or EMI!

 A CLOSER look...

The Tuskegee syphilis study

- Conducted between 1932–1972 by the US Health Service

- In Tuskegee, Alabama

- Followed up 600 African-Americans (two-thirds of which had contracted syphilis previously, one-third were disease-free)

- Aimed to study the natural course of the disease

- Failed to maintain good ethical standards

- Participants were not informed of their diagnoses or appropriately treated despite the discovery of penicillin as an adequate cure.

- Observed to be actively preventing participants from accessing syphilis treatment programmes.

- Multiple deaths ensued.

A CLOSER look...

The Nuremberg trials

- 1945–1956

- Series of 12 tribunals for war crimes.

- Held in Nuremberg, Germany post-Second World War.

- An example of one such tribunal is 'The Doctor's Trial'.

- In this trial, Nazi doctors were accused of human experimentation and the mass murder of prisoners of war.

- The trials led to the development of the Nuremberg Code (a group of research ethical principles to be adhered to in studies involving human experimentation).

- Examples of Nuremberg Code principles include obtaining voluntary consent, avoiding unnecessary physical and mental harm to participants and termination of the study by the researcher if continuation of the study is deemed to be of detriment to the health and safety of its participants.

A CLOSER look...

The Geneva declaration

- Developed in 1948 by the World Medical Association General Assembly.

- A revision of the Hippocratic Oath.

A CLOSER look...

The Helsinki declaration

• Developed in 1964 by the World Medical Association General Assembly.

• In Helsinki, Finland.

• Has undergone six revisions.

• Principles relating to conduct of clinical research

Chapter 8

Psychotherapy

Chapter 8
Psychotherapy

Freud

- Associated with classical psychoanalytical theory.

- Established structural and topographical models of the mind.

 A CLOSER look...

The topographical model of the mind

- **Unconscious**. Repressed unacceptable and unpleasant emotions. Primary process thinking.

- **Preconscious**. Mediates the unconscious and conscious.

- **Conscious**. Operates secondary process thinking. Reality-based. Enables individuals to communicate with the outside world.

The structural model of the mind

- **Id**. Pleasure principle. Primary process. Basic drives and instincts. Need for immediate gratification. Unconscious. Present since birth.

- **Ego**. Reality principle. Secondary process. Conscious. Mediates between id and reality. Present from 1 year of age.

- **Superego**. Moral conscience and ego ideal. Develops on resolution of the Oedipus complex.

Common terms used in psychoanalysis

Free association	Enabling individuals to speak freely without restriction.
Transference	When an individual unconsciously plays out and repeats past events in therapy with the associated emotion shifting focus onto the therapist.
Countertransference	Describes how the therapist feels about the patient.
Working through	Allows the patient to repeatedly play out past events in therapy with a view to resolving difficult issues.
Therapeutic alliance	Describes the relationship between the therapist and the patient.
Repression resistance	Difficulty of the patient in accessing the unconscious.

Common terms used in dream interpretation

Dream work	Turning the latent content into the manifest content
Latent content	Hidden, symbolic unconscious thoughts of the dream.
Manifest content	The content of the dream recalled by the dreamer.
Condensation	When a number of unconscious ideas and concepts are represented by a single image.
Diffusion	When a single unconscious impulse is represented by several images in a dream.
Parapraxes	'Freudian slips'. Error of speech or slip of the tongue said to reveal a repressed wish.

Common defence mechanisms

Subivided into mature, immature, neurotic and psychotic.

A CLOSER look...

Mature defences

- **Suppression.** Consciously 'putting on hold' unacceptable and unwanted memories, wishes and experiences.

- **Sublimation.** Process of channelling frustration or undesirable impulses into one without adverse consequences. *Example*: a pupil gets an F grade on his homework. Rather than direct his anger towards his teacher, he channels his frustration by agreeing to a game of hockey with his peers.

- **Humour.** Use of comedy to make an unpleasant impulse more tolerable.

- **Altruism.** To ensure that others welfare is put before one's own.

- **Anticipation.** 'Preparing for the worse'.

A CLOSER look...

Neurotic defences

- **Isolation.** Separating an idea from its associated affect.

- **Intellectualisation.** Focusing on facts rather than emotion ascribed to them.

- **Dissociation.** Characterised by temporary alteration of consciousness in an individual's sense of identity.

- **Displacement.** Redirecting emotions from one object or person to one that is less threatening.

- **Repression.** Unlike suppression which is conscious, repression is the unconscious process of excluding feeling and instincts.

- **Rationalisation**. Means of justifying what would otherwise be considered unacceptable behaviours.

- **Reaction formation**. Turning an unpleasant, undesirable impulse into its exact opposite.

A CLOSER look...

Immature defences

- **Acting out**. Unconsciously expressing an impulse to avoid being aware of the accompanying affect.

- **Regression**. Becoming child-like or sliding back into early developmental stages to avoid an undesirable conflict or impulse.

- **Projection**. Shifting one's own unacceptable, unacknowledged impulses onto others but perceiving the original impulse to have originated from them and not from the self.

- **Passive aggression**. Indirectly expressing aggression towards others.

A CLOSER look...

Psychotic defences

- **Splitting**. Splitting negative and positive impulses. Something is either viewed as wholly good or wholly bad. There is no in between. Common in those with borderline personality who may praise the nursing team but are overly critical of the medical team.

- **Denial**. Refusal to accept a threatening reality.

- **Projective identification**. Describes the behaviour of the recipient towards the object of projection.

Other important theorists

Carl Jung

- Proponent of analytical psychology
- Terms commonly associated with Jung include:
  - Personal unconscious
  - Collective unconscious
  - Persona
  - Archetypes
  - Animus
  - Anima
  - Complexes
  - Shadow.

Adler

- Proponent of individual psychology.
- Associated with inferiority complexes.

Melanie Klein

- Proponent of play analysis.
- Considered the paranoid–schizoid and depressive positions.

Winnicott

- Proponent of objects relation theory.
- Development of several concepts including holding, good-enough mother and transitional object.

Chapter 9

Psychopharmacology

Chapter 9
Psychopharmacology

Classification of psychotropic medication

Antipsychotics

Amisulpiride, Sulpiride	Substituted Benzamide
Aripiprazole	Arylpiperidylindole
Chlorpromazine, Promazine, Triflupromazine	Aliphatic Phenothiazines
Clozapine	Dibenzodiazepine
Droperidol, Haloperidol	Butyrophenones
Fluphenazine, Prophenazine, Trifluoperazine	Piperazine derivative
Olanzapine	Thienobenzodiazepine
Quetiapine	Dibenzothiazepine
Risperidone	Benzisoxazole derivative
Thioridazine	Phenothiazine (Piperidine derivative)

Antidepressants

Amitriptyline, Clomipramine, Dothiepin	Tertiary amine (tricyclic)
Imipramine, Trimipramine	

Amoxapine, Desipramine, Nortriptyline, Protriptyline	Secondary amine (tricyclic)
Citalopram, Fluvoxamine, Fluoxetine	Selective serotonin reuptake inhibitor (SSRI)
Paroxetine, Sertraline	
Duloxetine, Venlafaxine	Serotonin and noradrenaline reuptake inhibitor (SNRI)
Mirtazapine	Noradrenergic and specific serotonergic antagonist (NaSSA)
Moclobemide	Reversible inhibitor of monoamine oxidase A (RIMA)
Nefazadone, Trazadone	Serotonin antagonist and reuptake inhibitor (SARI)
Reboxetine	Noradrenaline reuptake inhibitor (NARI)

Hypnotics

| Zopiclone | Cyclopyrrolone |

Miscellaneous

| Bupropion | Aminoketone |
| | Dopamine reuptake inhibitor (DRI) |

Mechanism of drug action

This list is by no means exhaustive but aims to help you get your head around the detailed mechanisms of some of the commonly cited (in MRCPsych Exams) and trickier psychotropic medications.

Antidepressants

| Mirtazapine | 5HT2A antagonism |
| | Alpha-2 antagonism |

	Antihistaminic
	Anti 5HT3 properties
Trazadone	5HT2A/2C antagonism
	Alpha-2 blockade
	Alpha-1 and antihistaminic action

Antipsychotics

Amisulpiride	D2 and D3 antagonism
Aripiprazole	D2 partial agonist
	Partial 5HT1A agonist
	D2 antagonism
	5HT2A antagonist
Chlorpromazine, Promazine	Antimuscarinic
Clozapine	High ratio 5HT2/D2 blockade
	D1 mediated
	Potent D4 blockade
	5HT6 blockade
	Alpha-1 and Alpha-2 antagonism
	Anticholinergic (M4)
	Antihistaminic
	5HT3
Haloperidol	D2 antagonist
Olanzapine	5HT2A/D2 blockade
	Potent D4 and 5HT6 blockade
	Anticholinergic
	Antihistaminic
Paliperidone, Risperidone	5HT2A/D2 antagonist
	5HT2A antagonist
Quetiapine	'Hit and run' 5HT2A/D2 blockade
	Anticholinergic
Sulpiride	Pure D2 antagonist
Thioridazine, Thioxanthenes	D2 antagonist

Mood stabilisers

Carbamazepine	Sodium channel activation
GABApentin	GABA-A agonist
Lamotrigine	Na channel blockade
Lithium	Second messenger via inositol monophosphatase
Pregabalin	GABA analogue
Topiramate	GABA-mediated reuptake inhibitor
	Weak inhibitor carbonic anhydrase inhibitor
Valproate	GABA agonist/potentiation
Vigabatrin	GABA transaminase inhibitor

Anxiolytics

Benzodiazepines	Full agonist GABA-A complex
Clonazepam	Partial agonism benzodiazepine receptor

Miscellaneous

Bromocriptine	Dopamine agonism
Buprenorphine	Partial agonsim at opioid receptor
Bupropion	Dopamine and noradrenaline reuptake inhibitor
Buspirone	Partial HT1A agonist
Clonidine, Lofexidine	Presynaptic Alpha-2 agonism
Flumazenil	Antagonism at benzodiazepine receptor. Reversal for benzodiazepine overdose.

Types of neurotransmitter

Monamines	Acetylcholine
	Dopamine
	Histamine

	Epinephrine
	Norepinephrine
	Serotonin
Amino acids	GABA
	Glutamate
	Glycine
Small molecules (peptides)	Angiotensin II
	Cholecystokinin
	Endorphins

Types of receptor

There are two different types:

Ionotropic	Ligand gated
	Fast response
	Rapid increase in membrane permeability
Examples	Nicotinic acetylcholine receptors
	Glutamate receptors
	Serotonin 5HT3
	GABA-A
	Benzodiazepine
Metabotropic	G-proteins
	Phosphorylation mediated
	Via second messenger
	Slow response
Examples	All other 5HT receptors
	Noradrenaline
	Dopamine
	Muscarinic acetylcholine receptors
	Opioid mu receptors

Drug approval

Stage 1	Preclinical animal studies
Stage 2	Human trials for safety of drug – **phase 1**

| Stage 3 | Human trials for effectiveness against particular disease/condition – **phase 2** |

Stage 3   Human trials for effectiveness against particular disease/condition – **phase 2**

Stage 4   Human trials for superiority compared with similar drugs for similar disease/condition – **phase 3**

Stage 5   Post-marketing surveillance – **phase 4**

Drug metabolism

There are two phases involved in drug metabolism.

Phase 1 involves the processes of oxidation, reduction and hydrolysis whereas phase 2 involves conjugation.

Cytochrome enzymes

It is useful to have a fairly thorough understanding of the involvement of cytochrome enzymes in the metabolism of psychotropic medications. As demonstrated below this can stand to have a considerable impact on the concentration of psychotropic medication available in the bloodstream.

CYP1A2   **Substrates**: Clozapine, Duloxetine, Haloperidol, Olanzapine, tricyclic antidepressants

Inducers: smoking

Inhibitors: caffeine, Fluovoxamine

A CLOSER look...

Making sense of substrates, inducers and inhibitors

- Inducers will 'induce' (trigger) metabolism of the cytochrome enzyme which in turn will reduce the concentration of the substrate.

- Inhibitors will 'inhibit' (decrease) metabolism of the cytochrome enzyme which in turn will reduce the concentration of the substrate.

If we use CYP1A2 as an example:

Smoking will reduce the concentration of Clozapine due to increased metabolism (induction) via the CYP1A2 enzyme.

Conversely, caffeine inhibits the CYP1A2 enzyme resulting in reduced metabolism of Clozapine thus increasing its concentration.

CYP2D6	**Substrates**: Aripiprazole, Donepezil, Duloxetine, Fluoxetine, Galantamine, Mirtazapine, Paroxetine, Risperidone, tricyclic antidepressants
	Inhibitors: Duloxetine, Fluoxetine, Paroxetine
CYP3A4	**Substrates**: Benzodiazepines, Betablockers, Carbamazepine, Calcium Channel Blockers, Quetiapine, tricyclic antidepressants
	Inducers: Carbamazepine, Phenytoin
	Inhibitors: Fluoxetine, Nefazadone, grapefruit juice

Receptor-mediated medication side effects

Agitation	Alpha-2 blockade
	5HT2A/2C stimulation
	Dopamine reuptake inhibitor
Akathisia	5HT2A stimulation
	D2 blockade
Amnesia	GABA-A stimulation
	Anticholinergic
Anorgasmia	Alpha-1 antagonism
	5HT2A/2C stimulation
Anorexia (loss of appetite)	5HT2A stimulation
Delirium	Anticholinergic
Extrapyramidal side effects (EPSEs)	D2 blockade
Gastrointestinal side effects	5HT3

Hyperthermia	Antimuscarinic
Hyperprolactinaemia	D2 blockade, 5HT1A stimulation
Hypotension (postural)	Alpha-1 antagonism
Impotence	Alpha-2 blockade 5HT2A/2C stimulation
Insomnia	Alpha-1 mediated 5HT2A mediated
Sedation	Histaminergic
Sweating	Noradrenaline reuptake inhibitor Cholinergic mediated
Weight gain	Histaminic, 5HTc mediated

Medication-specific side effects

Antipsychotics

Amisulpiride	Hyperprolactinaemia ++
Aripiprazole	Well tolerated.
	Good side effect profile. Not associated with cardiac or extrapyramidal side effects. No associated hyperprolactinaemia or other endocrinological side effects such as weight gain or blood sugar imbalance.
Chlorpromazine	Photosensitivity Obstructive jaundice Weight gain Sedation EPSEs
Clozapine	Neutropenia Agranulocytosis Hypersalivation Sedation

Weight gain

Myocarditis

Constipation

Tachycardia, hyper/hypotension

Low incidence of EPSEs

Haloperidol   Extrapyramidal side effects

Olanzapine   Sedation

Postural hypotension

Weight gain

Anticholinergic side effects

Lower incidence of sexual side effects

Risperidone   Lower incidence of EPSEs and sedation

Hyperprolactinaemia common

Postural hypotension

Gastrointestinal side effects

Sulpiride   Hyperprolactinaemia ++

 A CLOSER look...

Antipsychotic side effects

- **Acute dystonia**. Onset within hours. Treatment: anticholinergics.

- **Akathisia**. Onset within weeks. Restlessness. Mediated via reduced D2 activity in basal ganglia. Treatment: beta blockers, benzodiazepines. Not anticholinergics.

- **Parkinsonism**. Onset within days. Mediated via reduced central D2 occupancy. Treatment with anticholinergics.

- **Tardive dyskinesia**. Onset within months. Mediated via supersensitivity D2 nigrostriatal pathway. Treatment: Clozapine. Not anticholinergics.

A CLOSER look...

Neuroleptic malignant syndrome

Symptoms: hyperthermia, rigidity, EPSEs, autonomic instability, fluctuating consciousness.

Investigations: Raised creatinine phosphokinase (CPK)

Treatment: Supportive management. Amantadine, Bromocriptine, Dantrolene, Diazepam, L-DOPA.

Mood stabilisers

Carbamazepine	Agranulocytosis
	Cognitive impairment
	Dizziness
Lithium	Hair loss
	Acne
	Psoriasis
	Tremor
	Metallic taste
	Polyuria/polydipsia
	Hypothyroidism
	Leucocytosis

A CLOSER look...

Lithium toxicity

- Symptoms: seizures, confusion, ataxia, coarse tremor, dysarthria.
- Treatment: alkaline diuresis.

Valproate	Weight gain
	Alopecia
	Polycystic ovaries

Important drug interactions

Carbamazepine and warfarin	Carbamazepine reduces warfarin levels
Carbamazaepine and oral contraceptive	Carbamazepine reduces oral contraceptive pill levels
Chlorpromazine and tricyclics	Increased plasma concentration of both.
Chlorpromazine and Clozapine	Lower seizure threshold
Lithium interactions	*See* Closer look box

A CLOSER look...

Lithium interactions

Lithium + Clozapine: increased risk of confusion and seizures.

- Carbamazapine, calcium channel blockers and typical antipsychotics: Lithium toxicity.
- Caffeine, Theophylline, Osmotic Diuretics reduce Lithium levels.

MAOI (monoamine oxidase inhibitors) + pethidine/atropine = fatal.

MAOIs + SSRIs	Serotonin syndrome
SSRIs + TCAs	Serotonin syndrome

A CLOSER look...

Serotonin syndrome

- **Symptoms**: agitation, hypomania, myoclonus, pyrexia and rigidity.
- When cross-tapering MAOIs and SSRIs, a two-week washout period is required. Due to the long half-life of fluoxetine, a longer washout period of five weeks is advised.

Tricyclic antidepressants + clonidine   Hypertensive crisis

Tricyclic antidepressants + MAOIs   Hypertensive crisis

**When prescribed MAOIs, individuals need to be careful with their diet to avoid offsetting a hypertensive reaction.

 A CLOSER look...

Cheese reaction (hypertensive crisis)

- Avoid red wine, cheese, yeast, pickled fish and liver.

- **Symptoms**: headache, hypertension, dilated pupils, chest pain, stiff neck, nausea and vomiting.

- **Management**: Chlorpromazine, Phentolamine.

Tricyclic Antidepressants + Warfarin   Increase warfarin levels, risk of bleeding.

Chapter 10
Psychopathology

Chapter 10
Psychopathology

This chapter simply provides an A–Z of common terms used to categorise and diagnose the patient's abnormal symptomatology, experiences and exhibited behaviours namely descriptive psychopathology.

Ambitendence	Alternating movements but never reaching desired goal.
Autocthonous delusion	Delusion occurring out of the blue.
Automatic obedience	Complying excessively with what is being asked.
Autoscopic hallucinations	Seeing an image of oneself: 'phantom mirror image'.
Catatonia	Rigid involuntary movement with increased tone of muscles at rest.
Circumstantiality	Delay in reaching the point. Talking around the topic. The intended outcome of the conversation is eventually reached, albeit slowly.
Concrete thinking	Inability to appreciate metaphorical speech. Taking things literally.
Déjà vu	Feeling as though events have occurred before.
Delusional atmosphere (mood)	The sense that 'something bad or significant' is about to happen.
Delusional memory	Belief over a false memory.

Delusional percept	A stimulus is normally perceived but with delusional meaning.
	Example: She saw a blue bus and immediately thought that the world would end today.
Derealisation	Feeling that your environment is unreal.
Depersonalisation	Feeling as though you are unreal.
Derailment	Disconnection between one thought and another, sequence of unrelated thoughts.
Echolalia	Repeating words uttered by others.
Echopraxia	Mimicking other's movements.
Extracampine hallucinations	Hallucinations experienced beyond the limits of possible sensory field.
	Example: I could hear her from the other side of the world.
Folie à deux	Shared delusion.
Functional hallucinations	Normal perception of one sensory modality triggers a hallucination in the same sensory modality.
	Example: everytime she heard the kitchen tap drip, she heard a faint whisper.
Fusion	Linking two unrelated thoughts.
Hypnagogic hallucinations	Hallucinations experienced upon going to sleep.
Hypnapompic hallucinations	Hallucinations experienced on waking.
Jamais vu	Feeling as though you have never experienced something which in fact you have experienced before.
Macropsia	Objects appear larger than they actually are.

Mannerisms	Odd, goal-directed movements.
Micropsia	Objects appear smaller than they actually are.
Mitgehen	Translates as 'to go with'. Moving limbs in the direction of the examiner's pressure.
Mitmachen	Individual is asked to resist attempts by the examiner to manipulate their limbs, but despite this allows the examiner to move them into abnormal postures.
Mutism	Refusal to speak.
Negativism	Refusing all passive movement.
Obstruction	Stopping movement mid action.
Over-inclusive thinking	Including into conversation irrelevant details.
Palinopsia	Visual image persists even after the stimulus disappears.
Perseveration	Repeating the same response despite other stimuli being presented.
	Example: the candidate is asked one question and gives their answer. The candidate is asked a second question but repeatedly responds with the answer to the first.
Posturing	Maintaining odd, abnormal postures.
Psychological pillow	A form of posturing whereby the patient can lie down with their head suspended in thin air, raised inches off the pillow.
Reflex hallucination	Stimulus in one sensory modality produces a hallucination in another field.
	Example: everytime she heard a bell ring, she experienced stomach cramps.

Stereotypes	Non-goal-directed movement.
Synaesthesia	Stimulus in one sensory modality is perceived as another.
	Example: She tasted the colour red.
Thought blocking	Cutting off during a trail of thought unexpectedly.
Thought insertion	Feeling as though thoughts are being 'put into one's head'.
Thought withdrawal	Feeling that thoughts are being taken away.
Verbigeration	Repeating words and sentences. Not goal-directed.
Waxy flexibility	Examiner is able to mould (as with wax) the individual's limbs into certain postures which are then maintained by the individual.

Chapter 11

Miscellaneous

Chapter 11
Miscellaneous

Eponymous syndromes

Capgras syndrome — Belief that a person close to you has been replaced by an imposter.

Cotard syndrome — Characterised by nihilistic delusion whereby the individual feels that they are dead or that bodily systems are shutting down or failing them.

Couvade syndrome — Sympathetic pregnancy affecting the husband's of pregnant women. Conversion.

De Clerambault's syndrome — Delusional belief by a woman that a man of high social status is in love with her.

Fregoli syndrome — Belief that a familiar individual is taking on various guises.

Othello syndrome — Pathological jealousy.

Culture-bound syndromes

Amok — Withdrawal, aggressive outburst and attack of others.

Dhat — Indian culture, somatic symptoms. Individual cites passage of semen in urine as reason for this.

Koro	South East Asia. Belief that penis is shrinking into abdomen and that death will ensue.
Latah	Malay women. Characterised by startle response, echolalia, echopraxia and coprolalia.
Pibloktoq	Occurs in Eskimos. Intolerance to cold, coprophagia (eating faeces), depression and echolalia.
Windigo	Affects North American Indians. Belief of practicing cannibalism.

Index